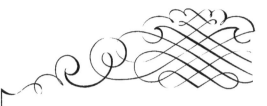

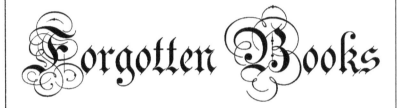

ISBN 978-1-397-32359-0
PIBN 11374462

1 MONTH OF
FREE
READING

at
www.ForgottenBooks.com

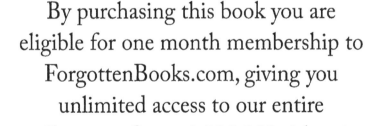

By purchasing this book you are eligible for one month membership to ForgottenBooks.com, giving you unlimited access to our entire collection of over 1,000,000 titles via our web site and mobile apps.

To claim your free month visit:
www.forgottenbooks.com/free1374462

English
Français
Deutsche
Italiano
Español
Português

www.forgottenbooks.com

Mythology Photography **Fiction**
Fishing Christianity **Art** Cooking
Essays Buddhism Freemasonry
Medicine **Biology** Music **Ancient
Egypt** Evolution Carpentry Physics
Dance Geology **Mathematics** Fitness
Shakespeare **Folklore** Yoga Marketing
Confidence Immortality Biographies
Poetry **Psychology** Witchcraft
Electronics Chemistry History **Law**
Accounting **Philosophy** Anthropology
Alchemy Drama Quantum Mechanics
Atheism Sexual Health **Ancient History**
Entrepreneurship Languages Sport
Paleontology Needlework Islam
Metaphysics Investment Archaeology
Parenting Statistics Criminology
Motivational

CAUSES

AND . . .

RECENT

TREATMENT

OF . . .

NEURASTHENIA

BY

JOHN D. QUACKENBOS

A. M., M. D.

CAUSES AND RECENT TREATMENT

OF

NEURASTHENIA

BY

JOHN D. QUACKENBOS, A. M., M. D.

Fellow of the New York Academy of Medicine
Member of the New York Academy of Sciences
Fellow of the New Hampshire Medical Society

PRESENTED AT THE ANNUAL MEETING

OF THE

NEW HAMPSHIRE MEDICAL SOCIETY

MAY 25th, 1897.

Compliments of RIGAUD & CHAPOTEAUT
With permission of the Author.

MORRISON PRINT,
43 Broad Street, New York.

CAUSES AND RECENT TREATMENT OF NEURASTHENIA.

BY JOHN D. QUACKENBOS, M. D., NEW YORK.

A paper presented at the Annual Meeting of the New Hampshire Medical Society, May 25th, 1897.

Neurasthenia or *Nervous Exhaustion*, the so-called "American disease," is not modern, but belongs to that category which the man of wisdom had in mind when he remarked, "There is no new thing under the sun." It has afflicted the human race from the beginning of history. Indeed, if we believe Milton, before man knew what suffering is, the arch-enemy of our kind, after that "dubious battle on the plains of Heaven," and the fall to that state where "peace can never dwell, hope never comes," tasted to the full the agony of the neurasthenic:

"Me miserable! which way shall I fly, infinite despair?
Which way I fly is Hell; myself am Hell;
And in the lowest deep, a lower deep
Still threat'ning to devour me opens wide,
To which the Hell I suffer seems a Heaven."

A political outcast, object of the ridicule of a dissolute court, shattered in health and in fortune, blind and helpless, and not a stranger to that ingratitude which Shakespeare described as sharper than a serpent's tooth—John Milton seems to me to have put into the mouth of Satan an accurate description of his own mental suffering.

As I glance over the biographical records of the past in search of evidence confirmatory of Arndt's assertion that neurasthenia has been recognized for thousands of years, I find the Greek and Sanscrit classics replete with instances of emotional exhaustion; melancholia from disappointment in love; piqued women like Lesbian Sappho, who flung themselves from Leucadian capes; sexual neurasthenics and perverts; with a few overworked cases like the scholastikoi, or befuddled book-worms, that figure in the "Facetiæ" of Hierocles. The typical neurasthenic figure in Semitic history is Job, with his malassimilation, his auto-infection, and his cell-exhaustion from mental strain. And the Lord, his physician, gave him the advice we are so ready to extend to the modern neurasthenic, "Gird up thy loins like a man."

Perhaps the most marked case of neurasthenia in antiquity is that of Mæcenas, who certainly affords a conspicuous instance of nervous prostration. According to Seneca (de Provid., iii: 9), he was an insomniac. Horace (Odes, ii: 17) pictures him as a hypochondriac, and Pliny (vii: 51) as troubled with a continual restlessness. In fact, he exhibited all the stigmata of degencration, including what seems to be effemination, if not androgyny, inasmuch as he dressed like a woman (Seneca Epistles, 114), and was noted for his want of manliness. The accounts of his life indicate that his neurasthenia was the result of the same causes that operate to-day to produce the disease.

Although thus not an American affection in its origin, neurasthenia is peculiarly American in its distribution— the rush and tear and overwork, the emotional excitement connected with failure and success, the slavery to social obligations and pleasures, so characteristic of American women, sufficiently accounting for its wide spread existence in this country. American fashionable

4

and business life is a continuous nerve-storm. Nor again is it peculiarly the rich man's disease, for it afflicts as frequently the poorer classes, on whom fall so heavily the burdens incident to battle with the world. I have been surprised at its prevalence among the resident population of this state, especially as a sequel of the grip or influenza, of typhoid and of the zymotic diseases generally (toxic neurasthenia), and in its climacteric phase with the native women, broken down by a life-long domestic service or by excessive child bearing and lactation. The symptoms are generally misunderstood, and the condition is improperly treated, or regarded with suspicion, indifference, or ridicule. It is not my purpose to dwell upon the symptoms of neurasthenia—the paræsthesias and hyperæsthesias; the asthenopia and atonic voice; the deficient thirst (all neurasthenics are hydrophobiacs, with desiccated nerves); the constipation and fermentative dyspepsia, with their accompanying intoxications; the oxaluria and uricacidæmia; the vertigoes and helmet headaches; the loss of vaso-motor tone; the sensitiveness to noises, vibrations, and jars incident to existence in a land of electric and steam cars, of jostling crowds, clanging factories, and crowded streets and stores; the failure of sexual power and pleasure in the sexual act; the intractable sleeplessness; the agonizing tension as though under some frightful brain pressure; the sickening oppression about the præcordia (præcordialangst); the morbid fears, especially monophobia (fear of solitude) and anthropophobia (fear of society); the dread of responsibility; the indecision and *folie du doute;* the fixed conviction of incompetence and uselessness; and the delusional mental state, with its imperative conceptions. I need hardly picture the climax of this condition, at which faith and hope and love are, as Milton said, turned to Hell; at which Christian principle at last relaxes its hold on the tortured soul, and the sufferer of woes indescribable buries his agony in a self-sought grave.

There is a distinct line of demarkation between this state and insanity, in that it is amenable to curative treatment. The neurasthenic, if properly dealt with, may, in the great majority of cases, be saved, restored to comparative health, and made a useful and happy member of society again.

Permit me now briefly to discuss the direct physiological cause of the neurasthenic condition, and acquaint you with the treatment which I consider philosophical, and which I have found invariably to a greater or less degree successful.

Neurasthenia is a depraved state of the nervous system, caused by malnutrition of the nerve elements, through the abnormal disassimilation of the complex phosphorus-bearing nerve substances.

A nerve cell is a cell-body under control of a nucleus, and provided with branches or processes, the principal one of which, regarded as the true outgrowth of the cell, is called a *neuron*. It is the seat of ceaseless metabolic change, conditioning the replenishment of the contained phosphorus-bearing substances that represent so much stored or potential nerve energy, and that are transformed and consumed in the evolution of such energy.

Physiologists believe that the passage of nerve impulses alters the *osmotic* powers of the cell wall toward the surrounding plasma, and that by *endosmosis* and *exosmosis* the nutritive exchange takes place. The dense network of capillaries environing the cells indicates that they are the centres of this nutritive metabolism. In neurasthenia, not only are the nutritive properties of the cell-encircling plasma altered by auto-intoxication, the poison of infectious diseases, or by alcoholism, cocainism, morphinism, etc., but in some instances, through the action of the same causes, the

6

cells appear measurably to have lost the power to appropriate what limited amount of nourishment may be present. In either case, the cell-bodies are more or less starved and their energy-projecting powers correspondingly impaired.

No doubt the commonest cause of this cell-exhaustion and consequent impoverishment of nerve force—*the cause of the cause of neurasthenia*—is the intemperate exercise of the intellectual faculties and the excessive indulgence of the emotions and passions. I believe emotional unrest to be a far more prolific cause than labor dissociated from irritation and anxiety. The greater number of neurasthenics are unmarried persons, the operative causes in single men being the excitements connected with sexual and alcoholic excesses and with gambling; in single women, the harrassing struggle for bread. Sexual abstinence is in itself a predisposing cause of neurasthenia; but sexual excesses and irregularities are an every-day active cause. Sexual intercourse, naturally and temperately used, is a nerve sedative and tonic; intemperately or unnaturally indulged in, a nerve irritant and drain. It is not the passage of semen, nor the secretion of mucous fluid by the glands of Bartholini, that does the mischief; but the repeated orgasm or reflex act of ejaculation, which, like an epileptic convulsion, implies a nerve shock, and which exhausts the protoplasm and shrinks the nuclei of the cells as do electric discharges through them.

In some ill-understood manner, all such abuses produce cell-degenerating toxines not apparent to the microscope or appreciable by chemical anaylsis. Whatever, by prolonged or excessive action, enfeebles the system, must exhaust the cell-bodies faster than they can reproduce themselves. A sufficient amount of nutritive material is not floated to the centres of abnormal cell-activity to compensate for the extra demand made upon

7

them, nor are the waste products removed as speedily as is consistent with health and safety. And what are the results? Malnutrition and auto-intoxication.

When we exercise our muscles merely for the sake of pleasure, the amusement is called play. When we similarly exercise eye and ear, the amusement is known as æsthetic feeling. The first is active; the second passive. In each case pleasure accompanies the activity of well-nourished and underworked organs. On this principle human health and happiness hang—well-nourished and underworked cells—a normal amount of activity in the terminal nerve organs of the cerebro-spinal nervous system. But let certain nerves be called upon to perform an excess of work, and painful feeling results. Note the effect of dynamo-generated electric light upon the eye. Those who use the incandescent lamps for reading may refer the massive pain and feeling of irritation in the eyeball that follows an evening's work, to the imperceptible unsteadiness in the white-hot filament of carbon. This light really pulsates—rises and falls with the passage of each commutator bar under the brushes in the dynamo. If the engine be slowed down, the fluctuations become visible; but whether they are consciously appreciated or not, the nerve fibres in the retina must certainly respond, and the eyes become wearied; because, although the optic fibres are renewed seventeen times a second in order that we may learn so much and so unremittingly of the world about us, the destructive metamorphosis here is in excess of repair. In like manner, in all normal cerebral and nervous activity, we have constantly induced partial fatigues, followed by partial stimulations. In over use, the reparative processes are distanced by destructive metamorphosis; nutritive regeneration is unable fully to restore the wasted substance of the nerve-organs; and where the hours of sleep are invaded to meet the demands of a growing business or an imperious ambition, these nerve-organs rapidly lose the power of regeneration and become incapacitated for the fulfillment of their functions. Hence the morbid impulse to ingest more food than can be oxidized; hence the phosphaturia and uricacidæmia, the indigestion, and the neurasthenic liver. I hold that these are the effects of nerve starvation, not the origin of it; and here the mistake is made by many practitioners who treat merely the symptoms, forgetful to remove the causes that give rise to the symptoms. The nerve exhaustion primarily acts to produce the oxaluria, uricacidæmia, gastric and intestinal dyspepsia, prostatic neuroses, irritable and depressing sexual functions, muscular insufficiencies of the eyes and general asthenopia, præcordialangst, insomnia, and cardiac breakdown; and these results react as causes to perpetuate the nerve exhaustion. In neurasthenia, effects immediately assume the role of causes, and hence the danger of error in treating the disease.

You ask whether the microscope has revealed any deviation from the normal in cells that are in a condition of pathological fatigue. We all know from autopsies the toxic effects of infectious and acute inflammatory diseases in shrinking the nuclei and curtailing the processes of cephalic and cornual cells. We also know from experiments made on the lower animals that at the end of a day of active toil, the nuclei appear small and shrunken, but after a night of rest the cells are turgid with large, well rounded nuclei. Hence we certainly are justified in the inference that the cell-bodies of neurasthenics exhibit peculiar signs of defective nutrition. Says Gray: "The same cell that can become organically altered can become functionally altered; or the pathological alteration which we call general paresis, poliomyelitis, or peripheral neuritis, may have its functional analogue in cerebral, spinal, or peripheral neurasthenia, with this difference, that the cell which is originally altered in its molecular constitution cannot be made to return to the normal so readily as the functionally impaired cell."

Dr. Ira Van Gieson, the state pathologist of New York, writes me, under date of April 2, that his opinion coincides with my own, viz.: that there is some measure of toxicity degeneration in the nerve cells of neurasthenics. But the demonstration of such changes must involve very great difficulties, as well on account of the enormous amount of territory in the cortex to be examined, as by reason of the difficulty of obtaining neurasthenic material for autopsy purposes. As yet no work has been done along the new lines of research in the application of the methods and principles of modern cellular biology to the study of neurasthenia. However, treatment on the theory of cell-exhaustion and the practicability of cell-feeding has been the most successful. I believe that if the rest be made long enough, the food stimulating enough, the sleep regular, the change of employment judicious, and all worry removed, most cases of neurasthenia may be greatly improved, if not entirely cured. The trend of this treatment is wholly in the line of *nutritiou and direct stimulation af the spinal cord.*

Chemistry has demonstrated the presence of a phosphorus-bearing substance in the nerve cells. This is known as lecithin (*lecithos*, literally yolk of an egg), a hygroscopic white, waxy solid, composed of carbon, hydrogen, nitrogen, *phosphorus*, and oxygen. It is a constituent of every cell in our bodies, but especially characteristic of those that make up brain and nerve substance. Chemically, lecithin is a *phospho-glycerate of neurin*—neurin constituting the albuminous basis of nerve tissue and occuring in the gray granular vesicular nervous matter and in the white fibrous nervous matter. Lecithin is found also in pus, in the white corpuscles, and in semen. In combination with cerebrin, it constitutes protagon, the principal form in which it is met with in the brain. Life depends on the presence of healthy lecithin. Neurasthenia is due to a diminished amount or a reduced quality of this phospho-glycerate. Hence the philosophy of administering a *phospho-glycerate of lime** in conditions characterized by defective nutrition of nerve and brain cells, which means a diminution of phosphorus in the cerebral and nervous matter. Attention was first called to the value of phospho-glycerate of lime in the treatment of neurasthenia by Dr. Albert Robin, before the "Académie de Médecine" of Paris, as recently as 1894, and Chapoteaut's French preparations began to be used by a few American physicians in 1895. Phospho-glycerate of lime has been found rapidly to restore to the system the phosphorus eliminated in excess through the urine, and was proved by Robin to diminish the excretion of incompletely oxidized phosphorus there present and indicative of pathological waste. It supplies the exhausted and enervated cells with phosphorus in a state of combination essentially the same as that naturally contained in them—an organic or physiological phosphorus, as it were—readily assimilable, and thus differing from the mineral phosphorus of the popular syrups of the hypophosphites and the ordinary unassimilable phosphate of lime. Its administration at once stimulates nutrition, promoting metabolism, and hastening the rapid tissue interchange which constitutes health. In sexual neurasthenia and the impotence of old age, the effect of the phospho-glycerate is especially marked. Sexual energy and the pleasure connected with the sexual act are quickly restored. I have notes of cases in which persons upward of seventy years of age regained under its influence the full powers of

* Sometimes written glycero-phosphate or glyco-phosphate of lime.

middle life.   Treatment of neurasthenia with phospho-glycerate of lime is the treatment that ignores reflexes and directly addresses the seat of the disease.

It would be trespassing on your time to retail here the ideas of treatment that are to be found in the standard text books.   With me they have too often proved un-satisfactory.   But I will briefly outline for your consider-ation the method that I follow.   I administer four to eight grains of the phospho-glycerate of lime in capsules with each meal, and continue this treatment unremittingly for a year, or until cure is effected, not expecting results that are apparent and gratifying to the patient until after three or four weeks of medication.   There are cases characterized by marked physical depression in which I prefer *the wine* * *of the phospho-glycerate of lime*—a sherry-glassful before meals.   Its action is immediate, and the slight stimulation due to the alcohol seems to be main-tained by the absorption of the phospho-glycerate with the food.

With the phospho-glycerate of lime at meal time, I combine a fortieth or fiftieth of a grain of strychnia, to promote the nutrition of the cord ; and this I continue for a month, then drop it for a week or two, and resume for another month.   In connection with this nerve feed-ing, I seek to accelerate, through the several channels of exit, the elimination of waste products and toxins. At every relapse, I give calomel; during the treatment, cathartic mineral waters before breakfast, in sufficient quantity to produce a laxative and not a daily cathartic effect.   I insist on the drinking of plenty of water, hot or cold, between meals, to keep the kidneys flushed, Vichy, if obtainable, preferred.   Stimulate the skin with a daily bath and rub-down, and where the patient can endure the shock, the cold douche to the spine on rising. Keep the mind interested in something.   Physicians are

* 50 centigrammes to the fluid ounce.

12

finding out that the occupation cure is preferable to the rest cure, which is responsible for an overproduction of confirmed invalids. Dr. Skene's latest conclusion is to the effect that most neurasthenic women are either disappointed spinsters or spoiled wives who have been improperly treated—or rather cosseted—for trivial disorders. For these he recommends the exercise cure, preeminently dancing and horseback riding, not the bicycle. And yet the bicycle has been recommended by Hammond, and *is*, as we all know, a most useful adjuvant in the treatment of nervous disease.

Where insomnia persists, sleep must be induced by artificial means. This is of supreme importance, for in normal sleep the changes throughout the nervous system are recuperative, and the loss of sleep is fraught with greater damage to nerve substance than starvation through overwork or under-feeding. It is through physiological sleep, where there is no opportunity for nervous discharge, that the system attains its highest degree of efficiency, and becomes possessed of an unusual quantity of potential energy, which physicists ingeniously define as capacity for performing work.

Some neurologists contend that it is better for the patient to lie awake night after night than to resort to hypnotics, but this is not true. If sleep be induced by suitable hypnotics, it is seldom necessary to administer them two evenings in succession. Where all drugs fail, hypnotism will succeed, and the current of the disease may be changed by post-hypnotic suggestion.

The psychical treatment consists in securing the confidence of the patient and making him believe that he is curable—that there is a time ahead when he will be entirely well again ; but that he must have faith and not be discouraged at the chain of relapses which mark the course of the disease. When he gains a higher plane, he should be instructed to obey strictly the laws of work and play and diet that he has discovered to be good government for him.

If the case be one of traumatic neurasthenia, commouly called "railroad spine," with indisposition, sometimes inability, to use mind or muscles, it is our duty to discourage litigation. Worry thereabout, brooding over trouble, transforms the neuroses into a cortex habit, and the patient may become an invalid for life.

If anything is to be added to this treatment, it is exercise within the limits of fatigue, any kind of riding or rowing preferred to walking ; fresh air at an altitude not exceeding two thousand feet ; a nutritious and easily digested diet, in which phosphorus-bearing grains play an important part, and red wines rich in phosphate of iron are judiciously used ; and finally, the most conscientious observance of the old Greek law—*Meden agan* or *Nothing too much.*

16

PURE STRONTIUM SALTS.

(PARAF-JAVAL).

The Bromide and Lactate are made by the Paraf-Javal process and are free from every trace of Barium.

The investigations of Dr. Laborde communicated to the French Academy of Medicine, prove that the chemically pure Strontium salts (Paraf-Javal) have certain advantages which are not found in those of Potassium and Sodium.

Since their introduction in 1891, the Bromide, Iodide and Lactate have been the subject of a great number of communications on the clinical results observed in every country, and they may be now looked upon as belonging to our most valuable modern therapeutic agents.

BROMIDE.

The Bromide is recommended by Féré, Constantin Paul, Dujardin-Beaumetz and Coronedi, as a sedative, analgesic and anti-emetic, and has been found specially useful in all nervous affections and epilepsy, as well as in suppressing the most incoercible cases of vomiting of pregnancy. The same happy effects have been observed in gastritis, hysteria, acute gastric catarrh, the chronic glandular gastr·tis of Brunton, chronic lead poisoning, and the septicæmia consequent upon abortion.

As a gastric analgesic in vomiting of nervous origin, it acts by diminishing the excitability of the nerve centres and then of the nerve endings in the stomach. It relieves nervo-gastric irritation and controls morbid gastro-intestinal fermentation, without causing depression or any toxic symptom.

17

IODIDE.

The Iodide has proved very valuable in the treatment of Scrofulous, Rheumatoid and Cardiac disorders and Syphilis.

The *Standard Solution* of Iodide of Strontium (Paraf-Javal) contains 30 grains to the fluid ounce, and the *Standard Solution* of the Bromide of Strontium (Paraf-Javal) ℨ i to the fluid ounce. As a general rule the Iodide and Bromide are indicated in the *same cases* and in the *same doses* as the Potassium and Sodium preparations. The eruptions however, caused by the Potassium salts are not produced.

LACTATE.

The Lactate is indicated in certain forms of diabetes and is found to diminish the amount of albumin excreted in Bright's disease, and in the parenchymatous and rheumatical nephrites of nephritic and scrofulous patients, as well as in the albuminuria of pregnant or recently delivered women. Dose : a teaspoouful of the *Standard Solution* (ℨ i to the fluid ounce) three times a day.

The Strontium Salts (Paraf-Javal) and their Standard Solutions, are made only in the laboratories of

RIGAUD & CHAPOTEAUT, Paris,

U. S. AGENTS: E. FOUGERA & CO., N. Y.

APIOLINE.

(CHAPOTEAUT).

NOT TO BE CONFOUNDED WITH SO-CALLED APIOL.

The true active principle of parsley
dispensed in capsules of 20 centigrammes.

M. Chapoteaut has adopted a process for the extraction of the true active principle of parsley, which is a thick reddish liquid boiling at 275° C. (527° F.) specific gravity 1.113, called Apioline.

Professor Laborde's * exhaustive study of the action of Apioline, indicates that it stimulates the intestinal and genital vaso-motor system and hence has a decided action on the utero-ovarian reproductive apparatus.

Apioline is indicated in spasmodic and congestive dysmenorrhœa and is decidedly the most reliable agent we know of in amenorrhœa.

DOSES:

In Amenorrhœa.—One capsule 2 or 3 times a day during the week preceding menstruation ; continue the dose for 2 days when the flow is established.

In Dysmenorrhœa (spasmodic or congestive).—One capsule twice daily, immediately before and during the menses.

Dispensed in original packages containing 24 capsules only.

Apioline is made in the laboratories of

RIGAUD & CHAPOTEAUT, Paris,

U. S. AGENTS: E. FOUGERA & CO., N. Y.

* J. LABORDE, directeur des travaux physiologiques à la Faculté de medicine de Paris.—*Tribune medicale, January 8, 1891.*

Imitations and

Substitutions!

We take this opportunity of stating, that we cannot be held responsible for disappointing therapeutical results, **unless physicians insist upon druggists using only those preparations made in our laboratories.**

RIGAUD & CHAPOTEAUT.

We are actively introducing to the profession, so
ties for which we are agents, and believe you will sh
for the same.

The Jobbers throughout the United States an
stocks and the prices are given below.

CYPRIDOL Capsules, (Bottles of 50,)   -   -   -   !
   "   Injection, (6 tubes for hypodermic use,)   - $
HYDRARGYNE (Antiseptic leaves, 10 in a packet,)   -   !
CEREVISINE (in 3 ounce Bottles,)   -   -   -   -
COLCHIFLOR Capsules, (Bottles of 30,)   -   - $
GRIMAULT'S Indian Cigarettes,   -   -   -   -

E. FOUGERA & CO., 26, 28, 30 N. William S

cly introducing to the profession, some new speci...
are agents, and believe you will shortly have ca...

throughout the United States and Canada ho...
are given below.

(Bottles of 50.)	$6.00 per doz.	
...ion, (6 tubes for hypodermic use.)	$16.00	"
Antiseptic leaves, 10 in a pocket.)	$3.00	"
3 ounce bottles.)	$8.00	"
...upaine, (Bottles of 50.)	$12.00	"
...dian Cigarettes.	$4.00	"

CO., 26, 28, 30 N. William St., N.Y. CH...

CPSIA information can be obtained
at www.ICGtesting.com
Printed in the USA
BVHW061024180219
540537BV00015B/739/P